SIRTFOOD DIET 2.0:

THE NEW GUIDE TO WELLNESS AND HEALTH

The new edition of June 2021 to lose weight fast with the "Skinny Gene". Includes Sirt Recipes for an active life and body health.

TABLE OF CONTENTS

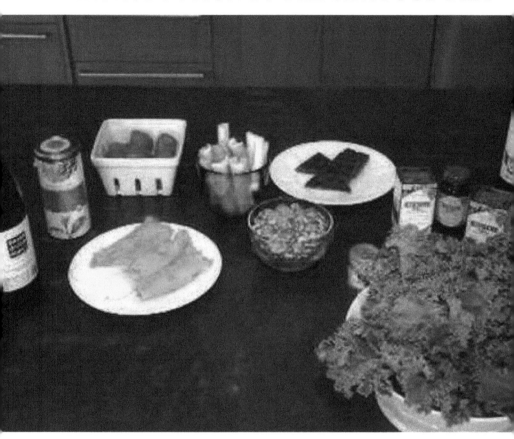

Sirtfoods are a recently discovered group of nutrient rich foods which seem to be able to 'activate' the body's skinny genes (also known as sirtuins), in much the same way as fasting diets do, with the same range of benefits, but without the common downsides of fasting diets, such as hunger, irritability and muscle loss.

By eating a diet rich in Sirtfoods, it is claimed that participants will lose weight, gain muscle, look and feel better and maybe even live a longer and more healthy life.

The Sirtfood Diet was created by nutritionists Aiden Goggins and Glen Matten. They were so interested by the potential of Sirtfoods, they created a diet based around maximising Sirtfood intake and mild calorie restriction. They then tested this diet on participants from an exclusive London gym and were amazed by their findings. Gym members lost an average of 7lbs in the first 7 days, despite not increasing their levels of exercise. Not only did the participants lose a substantial amount of weight, but they also gained muscle (usually the opposite happens when dieting) and reported significant improvements in overall health and well-being.

What sounds like a snack lifted straight from a sci-fi movie, a 'sirtfood' is actually a food high in sirtuin activators, says nutritionist Rob Hobson. Sirtuins are a type of protein which protect the cells in our bodies from dying or becoming inflamed through illness, though research has also shown they can help regulate your metabolism, increase muscle and burn fat, hence the new 'wonderfood' tag. Sirtfoods are mostly plant-based and high in antioxidants that help trick your body into burning fat at a higher rate. It's called Sirt because it includes eating foods that are high in sirtuin activators, defined as seven proteins found in the body that regulate metabolism, inflammation, and the longevity of cells.

THE BASIC AND ESSENTIAL PRINCIPLES YOU NEED TO KNOW ABOUT WEIGHT AND FAT LOSS

These days almost everyone is concerned with losing weight or more importantly losing fat. I am asked more questions about this topic than all others and it is an obvious source of confusion for many people. The problem is there are many different opinions about the best way to lose fat and most have at least some truth to them.

One popular strategy suggests concentrating on the percentage of calories from fat that you burn during the exercise. This leads to recommendations for exercising at a particular intensity/heart rate, which is often called the fat burning zone. This sounds like a good way to figure out how to exercise for maximal fat burning, but when you exercise to burn the highest percentage of fat, you end up burning fewer total calories, because the exercise intensity is too low.

Another common strategy is to focus on the total number of calories burned during your workout instead of the actual fat calories. This is recommended because unless you burn more calories throughout the day than you consume, you will never lose fat, regardless of the percentage of calories you burn while exercising. This is true, but just looking at the number or type of calories burned while exercising never gives you the full story.

There are however other important factors that are often overlooked when determining how to exercise for optimal fat loss. First, some types of exercise, such as resistance training, may not burn a lot of calories during the actual workout, but your body will keep burning calories at a higher rate for many hours after you stop exercising. This increased calorie burning effect will vary depending on the duration, intensity, and type of exercise. As a result, it becomes very difficult to accurately determine how many calories are really burned due to your workout.

Fortunately, knowing how many calories or how much fat you burn while exercising is not as important as you might think. The real issue is how your workout affects your metabolism. Increasing your metabolism is by far the most beneficial thing you can do to improve long-term fat loss. Your metabolism is responsible for burning many more calories than exercise and if your main goal is fat loss, you should focus on increasing your metabolism as much as possible.

Increasing the body's metabolism is a complicated issue that is affected by genetics, exercise, nutrition, and a number of other lifestyle factors. Since this article is about exercise and this issue is too large to be properly addressed in this article, I will concentrate on a basic strategy to help improve your metabolism.

This strategy essentially has 2 main goals, preventing muscle loss and challenging your body. Muscle has a significant influence on your metabolic rate and every pound of muscle burns about 30 calories per day. If you stop doing exercises that stress your muscles, you will start losing muscle and your metabolism will slow down. Moderate to high intensity resistance training (weights, bodyweight exercises, etc.) is an ideal choice for this type of workout.

As a general rule, you should perform exercises that are difficult enough that you are unable to perform 15 reps; 6 to 12 reps per exercise is a good range. This may be more intense than your usual workout, but if you only have enough time for a short workout, it will be enough intensity to retain your current level of muscle. Also, since your exercise time will be short and the number of total sets will be low, you shouldn't have to worry about gaining muscle or bulking up. Bodybuilders have large muscles mainly because they perform an excessive number of sets, sometimes 20-30 per muscle group, not because they lift heavier weights.

The overall workout only needs to be 15-30 minutes long and you have some options as to how to design the workout. You can do 1 set of many different exercises, multiple sets of a few exercises or anything in between. With the increased intensity of the exercises, you probably won't want to exercise much longer anyway.

A higher percentage of leg exercises (squats, lunges, etc.) than usual is also suggested. This is because your largest muscles are in your legs and exercises that stress large muscles create a greater overall demand on the body and produce better metabolic improvements. Try for 35 - 40 % leg exercises if your workout is 30 minutes and around 50% if the workout is closer to 15 minutes. This approach will also maximize the number of calories burned during the workout and result in more calories being burned throughout the day.

If you would rather perform endurance activities (running, biking, etc.), you can apply the same principles of increasing the intensity to make the exercise more demanding. Perhaps the best method is to replace a constant intensity aerobic workout with a shorter interval training workout. This involves alternating between your normal pace and much more challenging pace. For example if you are a runner, you could alternate between running for 1 minute at your regular speed and sprinting for 30 seconds.

Regardless of which approach you take, you should feel about as fatigued at the end of your short workout as you do after a regular length workout. However, if you are not accustomed to more intense training, it is important to start out slowly and let your body adapt to the training. It is very important not to overdo it or push yourself too hard. You want to feel fatigued, but not run down or excessively sore. Also, even though the workout is short, you still need to warm up before the workout and stretch/cool down after you finish.

Keep in mind this strategy does not represent a complete well-rounded fitness program and is not intended to replace your existing program. It is especially useful during times when you may have a limited amount of time to exercise, such as while traveling and it is also beneficial for adding variety to your program. I chose this approach so people with different workout routines and overall goals could apply the strategy to their individual situations.

Look at your existing program and determine how to apply this information to benefit your most. In addition, be sure to remember that nutrition and lifestyle factors (sleep, stress, etc.) are always important too. You can have the best exercise program in the world and if you have bad nutrition and lifestyle habits you will still have a hard time losing fat

Before getting into any diet or workout program, you have to first understand how your bodily process works. The body has the ability to perform its daily function with a calorie maintenance level. The appropriate amount of calories enables you to walk around and maintain the inner bodily functions. Calories are the body's source of power. Without the proper quantity of calories, you'll feel sick.

The calories we need are from our drinking and eating habits. Weight does not go up or decrease when we eat the same number of calories fit for our daily requirements. Demonstrating this explanation: if your maintenance amount is 3000 calories and you eat an equal amount a day, you will not increase your weight. Weight increases when we consume more than our calorie maintenance level. The opposite, which is weight loss, occurs when we use up the daily maintenance level. We can also reduce calories by eating fewer from our everyday maintenance level. Hence, an individual with a 3000 calorie maintenance quantity should eat 2500 calories to reduce weight.

At this moment, you'd want to understand your calorie maintenance level. Your maintenance level is computed by using the Basal Metabolic Rate (BMR) of the Harris-Benedict Equation. The body's BMR is the quantity of calories you need to eat to maintain executing your daily responsibilities. How much activity you perform is considered when computing the calories you have to burn per day. You can look for everyday calorie maintenance level calculators online to understand what your body needs.

Now that you have comprehended the principle behind weight reduction, it's time to know the fundamental ways to lose weight. These 3 essential ways are all you require. The first is to work out. Exercise allows you to burn more calories. If you commit to your daily calories maintenance level, you'll end up losing that same amount. Thus, no weight change happens. But if you'd want to reduce weight, you'll have to engage in exercise that loses a greater amount from your calories maintenance level. With the past example, you will have to reduce additional 500 calories for weight loss.

Aside from exercise, you will also have to eat lesser of your daily maintenance amount. Those with a 3000 maintenance amount will have to sacrifice 500 calories and just eat 2500. A caloric deficit occurs as you give your body a lesser amount of the calories it needs for maintenance. Engaging in more of caloric shortages will give the body consistent weight loss.

The safest and most recommended method of weight loss requires both diet and exercise. Eating less calories and burning more calories gives the body a stability of what's gained and lost from your activities. It's been confirmed consistently that a healthy diet and workouts will give you quicker and long lasting weight loss results. Employing both methods are also the proper means and doesn't get in the way of your daily responsibilities.

Before you get into a workout routine or diet, you first must analyze your body's maintenance level. The analysis will be your form's adjustment into a better routine. Begin by eating your calorie maintenance level regularly for each day. Sustain such caloric consumption for 2 to three weeks. It doesn't have to be the same quantity of calories, as long as it is|comes very close. To ensure you're eating the appropriate quantity, weigh yourself once a week (before eating and on an empty stomach) in the day's beginning.

If you had a weight consistent for the two to 3 weeks, then you were able to eat the calories needed of your maintenance level. In order for you to reduce more weight, you must eat 500 less of your daily maintenance level per day. If your maintenance level is 2500, you will have to start consuming only 2000 calories a day.

Those who were unable to keep up their calorie maintenance level can still start a healthy weight reduction program. All you have to do is consume 500 less of your maintenance level and redo the body adjustment with the smaller calories quantity. If you were successful in eating the lessened maintenance level, then you must begom consuming minus 500 again of the initial amount.

It is important for one to ensure you do not lose the weight too fast. Reducing weight at a dangerous rate will compromise your well being. If you catch yourself losing three or more pounds each week regularly for some weeks in a row, then you'll have to make certain adjustments. The adjustment involves including 250 to 300 calories to your daily consumption. After which, you have to start watching your weight with the new quantity. Remember, you shouldn't just eat a smaller amount. You need to exercise to reduce enough calories for healthy weight reduction.

The prescribed weight reduction speed is around one to 2 pounds per week. Remember, reducing weight very quickly won't benefit your body. You have to maintain a loss speed that will continue to keep you fit. Your health is much more important than looking good. Our physique cannot catch up with very quick weight loss. In fact, it will simply change to stay alive if you quicken the procedure. Instead, body fat will be kept so it can catch up. Hence, you must only stick to shedding one to 2 pounds a week. If you're capable of doing so for one year, you'll eventually lose fifty to 100 pounds!

As we have already covered the calculations, it's time to get to the specifics. What type of meals should you be consuming? What must you avoid at all costs?

Let us start with the positive side. There's many delicious food out there that still allows you sustain and lose weight. Do not fall for fad diets that pretend low carbs or no fats will offer you the best outcome. These diets are only out to get profit from your desperation. A healthy physique requires all foods. You just have to balance them accordingly. The best experts to talk about meal choices with are physicians and nutritionists. They're give value for your money and are only looking out for your health.

A decent diet will entail the proper quantity of fats, carbohydrates, and proteins. An average healthy adult requires 30 % of their calorie intake to be from fat. So, if you consume 2000 calories daily, 400 to 600 calories will be from fat. Since 9 calories is found in 1 gram of fat, you'll have to consume 44 to 66 grams each day for the average person.

The best sources of fat are nuts, seeds, olive and canola oil, avocados, fish, fish oil, and flax seed oil formulas. Weight reducers should note that fat really does not make you "fat" if it comes from the healthy foods. Fat will not get in the way of your weight loss. It'll only contribute to your health and enhance your endurance. As long as you get your fat from the mentioned sources, you will not have to worry.

Another infamous food types for fad dieters is carbohydrates. It's advised that 50 % of your calorie intake are eaten from carbs. The conversion you have to recall: one gram of carbohydrates is four calories. Hence, someone who consumes 2000 calories per day will have to eat a thousand from carbohydrates. Thus, you have to consume

250 grams from carbohydrates a day. The healthies sources of carbs are fruits, sweet potatoes, beans, vegetables, oatmeal, and brown rice. In other words, eat complex carbohydrates and not the simple carbs. Simple carbohydrates are from sugary food like white rice, white bread, soda, and other highly processed foods.

As for protein, the recommended minimum daily amount is 0.8 grams for every kg of your body weight. To compute for this, divide your weight by 2.2 then multiply by 0.8. Since such is merely the minimum, people who participate in workouts should consume more than the computed amount. You can eat a bit more to assure your safety. The best choices of protein are turkey, chicken, fish, lean meats, eggs/egg whites, nuts, and beans.

Let us proceed to the meals you have to avoid. Most of these foods are obviously very bad for your well being. The basics to not eat are soft drinks, fast food, candy, cookies, crackers, cakes, pastries, and chips. Aside from these, don't eat food with Trans and saturated fat. Stay away from meals that have increased sodium and sugar levels. These meals||foods are usually where you get your extra calories. Aside from the added pounds, you will push yourself towards an unhealthy lifestyle.

Now that we have discussed the diet, it's time to discuss exercise. Working out is the best way for you to burn calories. Besides weight loss, it will also enhance||improve] your power, flexibility, and endurance. For the long run, it will also help you in preventing heart diseases and bone deteriorations.

There are 2 kinds of exercise for you to engage in: aerobic and anaerobic. Aerobic exercise is more renowned as the cardiovascular workouts. Cardio workouts enhance your cardiovascular endurance, done at a lasting pace in minimal to average forces. Cardio activities are walking, skating, jogging, swimming, biking, and elliptical machine activities. The most prescribed cardiology exercise is one that you enjoy and are eager to participate in habitually. Those who enjoy walking should do a daily walk. Bikers can continue with their pastime while swimming is perfect for water lovers. In terms of their time, the recommended schedule is thirty minutes. Those who can stillcarry on above it can still prolong. However, the thirty minutes is recommended for the average person. Do the cardio workout for about three to six days per week.

Anaerobic exercise puts focus on your muscle and stamina. These are typically weight training, calisthenics (like pushups), and using resistance machines. Anaerobic workouts burn you a notable quantity of calories. Although it is not as many as cardio workouts, they will enhance your stamina for the cardioexercises. It will also contribute very positive looks on your body. The increase of muscle will make you appear more toned and sexy. The advise speed of anaerobic exercises is between two to 4 times a week.

There are also some diet legends everyone must disregard. The first is the misconception consuming fat and carbohydrates makes you fat. Didn't we just state that fat and carbs are important to a person's health? You need these food types for your calories maintenance level. The next are those silly and useless one- meal diets. Just eating a small celery or cabbage soup will just kill you. Just eating one tiny food will not burn your fat. Your body will simply respond to the lack of food and sustain your current fat.

Another myth is that spot reduction workouts allow you to lose all your fats. Focusing on a single area is not the answer. This is because workouts focus on your muscles. If the muscles are sealed by fat, they will continue to be hidden. You'll have to reduce that fat for your muscles to show.

The most obvious fallacies are those products sold in infomercials. People do not lose their fat by relying on one sole product. Same goes with those ab machines. Such machines are only another instance of spot reduction. Any other fast or easy means to weight reduction is just out to get your money. You have to accept that weight loss entails perseverance and a large amount of your time.

If you want to invest cash for your weight loss, you should avail of a gym membership. Gyms have machines for both aerobic and anaerobic exercises. It is also a helpful motivator. You would not want to spend your money and not use that membership. You are also motivated by the individuals with you. Other means that will help you in weight reduction: digital food scale, treadmill, bike, elliptical machine, weights, tape measure, and a body weight scale.

In terms of your diet, you need to eat smaller foods more habitually. It is not recommended to eat one to three big meals a day. Instead, break it down into five to six small meals. Consume the meals every 2 to 3 hours. Another method to enhance your diet is to arrange your meals. Plan it on the beginning of the week and cook them early. This way, you are not bpunded by the fatty meals sold in restaurants or fast food places. You should also take your food with water. Drink it as you consume the meal. The water will make you full faster and stop you from consuming additional calories. Don't eat very fast. Your body will take some time to absorb that it is becoming full. Grind the food gradually and don't eat in a rush. If you eat too quickly, you'll consume more than your body actually requires.

Everybody wants to lose pounds. This is one fact that is manifestly supported by the countless weight loss programs in the market, together with the countless weight loss products, ranging from snack bars, powdered juices, shakes and even to slimming soaps and lotions! It can really be confusing making an attempt to understand which ones are for real and which of them are junk, especially when presented with all these information.

You Don't have To Practice Everything

It's not particularly necessary that you know wholeheartedly all the available diets out in the market. In fact, most of them can have conflicting principles. For instance, one would say that you need to eat a lot of little meals throughout the day, while another would say that you should only eat one large meal for the day and starve yourself till you start another day. Confusing isn't it? You need to research to find out which information is the real thing and which of them are not.

So, here are the necessary things you need to know about weight loss before you decide to endure any sort of diet program.

Losing Weight Is Not Instant

Although it might truly be glorious if you might shed weight straight away shortly after away shortly after employing a product, sadly you'd have to face the reality that losing weight is not an instant process. Don't be fooled with the countless diet programs and products that make 5-minute guarantees. Losing weight is rarely instant, unless you're undergoing liposuction surgery.

You should understand that it is a process that takes quite a long amount of time for it to be effective. There are really no shortcuts here. Unless you impose real discipline to yourself, in regard to eating healthy and living a healthy lifestyle, you would not lose weight on an everlasting basis.

Weight Loss Involves Activity

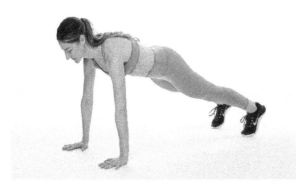

There are so many diet programs and each of them varies with their underlying beliefs. Watching what you eat is good. There is nothing wrong with that. However, you should keep in mind that food isn't the only factor that you should consider when trying to lose weight. Another crucial factor would be your body's activity.

If you need to shed some fat and make your diet effective, you should couple your food monitoring with the right exercise. Dieting want really work when you're living the life of a couch potato or you're simply in bed for the entire work when you are Living a couch potato or lifestyle will do you no good.

Starvation Is Not The Answer

Going on a hunger strike will not answer your fat issues. Believing in the popular belief that starving your body will make you shed pounds is a common mistake by many people. At first, this principle may make sense, it doesn't really work that simple.

If the body senses starvation, it automatically many folks. Initially, this as a signal for stress. When under stress, the body does automatic actions, such as production of hormones to negate this stress. In this situation, it produces more of cortisol, which is a vital hormone that excites fat production.

Additionally, your body will keep more water. When it starts water retention, this will definitely add to your body weight, since the body is especially composed from water.

Metabolism Varies

Metabolism is how fast or slow your body gets use from the food you eat and turn them into energy. You should understand that people do not have the body is especially consisting of metabolism. People have varied rates, and this may really affect how prone an individual is for gaining weight.

Generally, people with slow metabolism are prone to gain weight simply. Those with folk don't have the ones that may eat a lot yet still don't get fat. This is a good reason why eating what your chum eats within the day wouldn't necessarily lead you to ones that slim body that she has.

You may have different metabolic rates, which makes it okay for her to eat one entire box of pizza inside in the day without troubling of getting fat, while you get to eat all greens, that she has.

What you need to know about weight loss

In today's society, weight loss is becoming a more popular fad by the day. It has become the focus point of many conversations, the infamous New Year's resolution and the first worry before swimsuit season. However, most are shocked to realize that shedding those extra pounds are not as easy as first imagined. Many face problems because they are not educated about weight loss. In order to succeed, one must understand the concept behind achieving a healthier lifestyle.

What is Healthy Weight?

The most important goal should be to reach a healthy weight. Healthy weight is the weight ones body becomes when he/she eats a nutritious diet consistently, are physically active and balance the calorie intake with his/her physical activity. Being at this healthy weight can reduce of type two diabetes, high blood pressure, stroke, heart disease and certain types of cancer. To achieve a healthy weight, a physician should be consulted to create a weight loss program that is suited for the individual.

Difficulty with Losing Weight

If there are so many programs and techniques available, then why is losing weight so hard? Most weight loss is difficult because there are so many factors involved. Weight is influenced by genetics, metabolism, personal behavior, environment and culture. When considering all of these factors, it becomes a challenge to obtain the correct balance for weight loss. Most have better results when they shift to a healthier lifestyle than targeting weight loss alone. The main goal here is to develop healthier eating habits and combining them with regular physical activity. Creating healthy habits produces better long-term results than bouncing around from one diet to another.

Getting Started

Once the decision has been made to lose weight, it is important to maintain certain ideas throughout the process. The goal should be to achieve better health, not to lose so many pounds by the end of the week. Also remember that the change does not have to be made all at once.

Making small changes to one's daily routine can make significant improvements in his/her health. To be successful in making lifestyle changes, remember key points: don't diet, think about the relationship with food, slowly change eating habits, establish realistic goals and make physical a part of daily routine.

Losing weight is not only about appearance. It is about trying to create a healthier way of living. Weight control is a life-long effort and must be taken seriously. By implementing healthy changes and a positive attitude, one can be on the way to a successful weight loss.

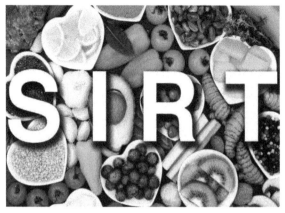

One major reason the sirtfood diet has exploded in popularity is due to its allowance of dark chocolate and red wine, as both items are considered sirtfoods. The claim is that by focusing on these foods, rapid weight loss will follow without decreases in muscle mass. A sirtfood dieter will begin their first week drinking green juice made of matcha green tea, lemon juice, parsley, celery, a green apple and arugula three times per week. After the first week, sirtfood dieters return to eating three meals per day made only with sirtfoods and will continue to incorporate these foods throughout the remainder of the diet.

The latest diet cleanse which has got the world raving about it follows a scientific approach to battle weight gain.

The diet popularises on the use of 'sirtfoods', which are some special foods which work by activating certain protein chains in the body, known as sirtuins. According to science, these antioxidant agents act as protectants that help slow down aging, boost metabolism and regulate the body's inflammation, hereby helping in fat loss.

Studies have also found that the sirtfood diet can help people lose up to seven pounds (3 kilos) in under a week's time.

As complex and scientific as this diet plan sounds, the diet encourages you to include some of the most commonly found kitchen ingredients as well as some indulgent foods. Some common foods allowed in this plan include foods like oranges, dark chocolates, parsley, turmeric, kale, and even red wine.

The diet, though considered to be a fad, focusses on maintaining a restrictive weight loss strategy one week. While the first three days makes you limit your calorie intake to 1000kcal (consuming three sirt food green juices and having a meal). The remaining days, you are allowed to increase your calorie intake to 1500kcal and have two meals a day (along with two sirtfood juices). Post this, the maintenance phase recommends you to eat up to three balanced foods rich in sirtuin, coupled with an effective workout strategy to lose weight, making it all the more sustainable.

Since it is rather restrictive in nature, many stay wary of the diet plan working in the long run. The diet restricts your calorie intake and can devoid you of other needed nutrients, so, it is not a long term, sustainable diet plan for weight loss.

There seems to be a growing number of celebrities and notable figures who've touted the sirtfood diet for their recent weight loss success. However, consumers must keep in mind that celebrities often have access to professional support when it comes to what they consume and any additional exercise regimens. Additionally, studies on the efficacy of this diet are slim. Granted, most foods listed are healthy whole food options and calorie restrictions which are automatically connected to some weight loss. The majority of foods listed have anti-inflammatory properties, high amounts of antioxidants and nutrients which are of course, beneficial. Medical experts warn though, that while quick weight loss is possible on such a diet, a majority of that initial loss will be water weight. It may also be risky for those who engage in moderate to high physical activity.

So how does the sirtfood diet works

The diet is split into 2 phases. Phase 1: the 7 day 'hypersuccess phase', which combines a Sirtfood-rich diet with moderate calorie restriction, and Phase 2: the 14 day 'maintenance phase', where you consolidate your weight loss without restricting calories.

PHASE 1 OF THE SIRTFOOD DIET

During the first 3 days, calorie intake is restricted to 1,000 calories (so, still more than on a 5:2 fasting day). The diet consists of 3 Sirtfood-rich green juices and 1 Sirtfood-rich meal and 2 squares of dark chocolate.

During the remaining 4 days, calorie intake is increased to 1, 500 calories and each day the diet comprises 2 Sirtfood-rich green juices and 2 Sirtfood-rich meals.

During phase 1 you are not allowed to drink any alcohol, but you can drink water, tea, coffee and green tea freely.

PHASE 2 OF THE SIRTFOOD DIET

Phase 2 does not focus on calorie restriction. Each day involves 3 Sirtfood-rich meals and 1 green juice, plus the option of 1 or 2 Sirtfood bite snacks, if required.

In phase 2 you are allowed to drink red wine, but in moderation (the recommendation is 2-3 glasses of red wine per week), as well as water, tea, coffee and green tea.

Phase two lasts for two weeks. During this "maintenance" phase, you should continue to steadily lose weight.

There is no specific calorie limit for this phase. Instead, you eat three meals full of sirtfoods and one green juice per day.

After the Diet

You may repeat these two phases as often as desired for further weight loss. However, you are encouraged to continue "sirtifying" your diet after completing these phases by incorporating sirtfoods regularly into your meals.

There are a variety of Sirtfood Diet books that are full of recipes rich in sirtfoods. You can also include sirtfoods in your diet as a snack or in recipes you already use. Additionally, you are encouraged to continue drinking the green juice every day. In this way, the Sirtfood Diet becomes more of a lifestyle change than a one-time diet.

How to do the sirtfood diet

Though the diet is often hailed as easy to follow thanks to the fact it includes red wine and dark chocolate, it's fairly strict in its guidelines.

The sirtfood plan relies on dieters restricting their calorie intake as well as eating a specific list of foods that are said to boost the metabolism.

The three-week plan involves an initial seven-day phase, followed by two weeks on phase two, AKA the "maintenance" phase.

One of the key components is a green juice which the founders call "rocket fuel", which followers of the diet have to make up to three times a day.

Sirtfood green juice recipe

- 75 grams (2.5 oz) kale
- 30 grams (1 oz) arugula (rocket)
- 5 grams parsley
- 2 celery sticks
- 1 cm (0.5 in) ginger
- half a green apple
- half a lemon
- half a teaspoon matcha green tea

Using a blender, juice all of the ingredients except for the green tea powder and lemon together, and pour them into a glass. Juice the lemon by hand, then stir both the lemon juice and green tea powder in.

This juice is important for phase one, which is designed to jump-start the weight loss. It involves restricting calories to just 1,000 a day (which is below the recommended daily intake).

Anyone following the plan would have three green juices per day plus one meal.

In the last three days of that initial week, the calorie intake increases to 1,500 a day, so you can add two more meals and have just two juices.

The recipes are all laid out in the official book, and include meals such as omelettes, salads and stir fries.

In phase two, dieters can then enjoy three sirtfood-rich meals and one sirtfood green juice a day, rather than watching the calorie count.

According to the founders, you should lose weight steadily throughout the plan.

A COMPLETE LIST OF HEALTHY AND DELICIOUS FOODS YOU CAN USE EVERY DAY

Losing weight can be challenging and there are so many choices, it's hard to sometimes decide what is healthy and what isn't. If you are looking for a sample of a food menu and need to know which foods are the best, then read on. Here you will learn about 10 foods which can be a dieter's best friend.

Low-Fat Cottage Cheese

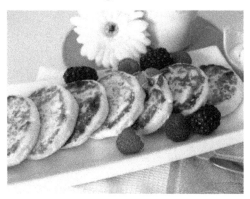 Low-fat cottage cheese can make a huge difference to anyone looking to shed a few pounds. It's low in fat, carbs and calories, while remaining high in protein. One-half cup of cottage cheese contains 15 grams of protein, nearly the same as 2 ounces of poultry, fish or cooked lean meat.

Cottage cheese is also very versatile, so if you don't care for the taste by itself, you can add in fresh fruit to sweeten it up a bit.

There are very few foods which are as healthy as cottage cheese. In addition to the aforementioned benefits, low-fat cottage cheese is also loaded up with Vitamin D and calcium, both which contribute to a healthy lifestyle.

Eggs

Eggs, like low-fat cottage cheese, are low in fat but high in protein. The fat that eggs do have is the right kind of fat. From the 5 grams of fat per egg, only 1.5 grams is saturated fat. If you're worried about cholesterol, don't be quick to dismiss eggs. The American Heart Association acknowledges that an egg a day is acceptable as long as you limit dietary cholesterol from other sources.

Many experts believe that saturated fats and trans fats have a bigger impact that dietary cholesterol in raising blood cholesterol. Eating an egg will make you feel fuller and curb your cravings for unhealthy snacks. Next time, why not reach for an egg instead of the chips.

Blueberries

By now, most people have heard about the many benefits of eating blueberries. Luckily, they are readily available and great for a mid-morning or a mid-afternoon snack when you need an energy boost. Blueberries contain load of antioxidants, which are thought to be important in reducing free radicals that can cause cancer and speed up the aging process.

According to researchers from the USDA Human Nutrition Center, blueberries are ranked number 1 in antioxidant activity when compared with 40 other fresh fruits and vegetables. Blueberries are perfect for the dieter because they are tasty, low in calories and high in nutrition.

Walnuts

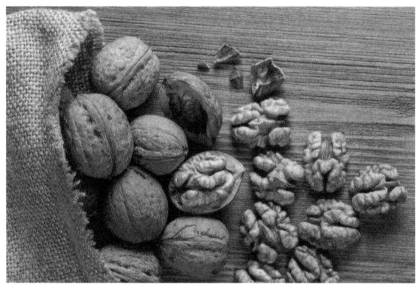

These are among the healthiest foods you can eat. Rich in fiber, magnesium, B vitamins and antioxidants like Vitamin E, they are also one of these best plant sources of protein. Walnuts have also been shown to lower LDL cholesterol (the bad kind).

Since nuts in general are high in fat, eating in moderation is the key. About 20 walnut halves (equivalent to 1.5 oz per day) is about the recommended serving of these tasty treats. Walnuts can be eaten alone as a snack or as toppers for salads, pasta, oatmeal and an almost infinite variety of dishes.

Spinach

Rich in vitamin C, fiber, carotenoids and iron, spinach is a nutritional powerhouse. Known to protect against cancer and heart disease, it's hard to beat this food. Spinach is tasty as a side dish (sautéed in a bit of olive oil and garlic) or as a foundation for a great salad. It's naturally low in calories and is high in flavor as well as nutritious.

Sweet Potatoes

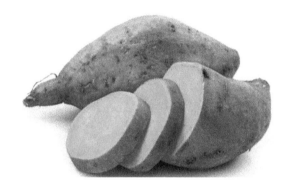

These naturally sweet vegetables are tasty and available almost year-round. Sweet potatoes have significant antioxidant qualities, in addition to being excellent sources of Vitamin A and Vitamin C. They also help fight inflammation and can help with diseases such as asthma and rheumatoid arthritis.

Sweet potatoes keep you feeling full for hours, which make the calories worthwhile. Sweet potatoes also have a low glycemic index, which means it breaks down slowly during digestion. It has been shown that lowering the glycemic load of the diet appears to be an effective method of promoting weight loss.

If you have a sugar craving, consider having a warm, baked sweet potato to curb your sweet tooth.

Watermelon

This tasty summer fruit is rich in potassium and Vitamin C. Watermelon is also a very good source of lycopene, which is preventative for a variety of cancers.

Watermelon is naturally low in calories, so it's the perfect no-guilt treat. If you're hungry for something fresh, juicy and sweet, watermelon is a great choice.

Salmon

Loaded with omega 3 fatty acids, this delicious pink fish can be served in a multitude of ways. Salmon contains a significant amount of the important omega 3 essential fatty acids, which are important in reducing unwanted inflammation and keeping our immune and circulatory systems healthy.

Salmon has plenty of protein, so it's filling and healthy to boot. Definitely a winning food!

Goji Berries

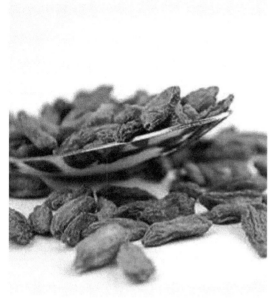

Although you might not be familiar with this tasty berry, it's so packed with vitamins, nutrients and protein, it is definitely a winning food.

These berries, also known as wolfberries, contain 18 kinds of amino acids, have more Vitamin C than oranges, more beta carotene than carrots and more iron than steak. Along with the ability to protect skin from sun damage they also help fight heart disease.

Goji berries can help in weight loss because they are high in fiber and also have a low glycemic index. They can be enjoyed as a snack by themselves, or in tea, juice, bars of cereal.

These berries are jam-packed with health benefits and are certainly worth a try.

Oatmeal

A large number of studies have shown that eating oatmeal can lower your cholesterol and help reduce your chance of heart disease. In addition, recent studies are showing that oatmeal may also help reduce the risk of type 2 diabetes. For those reasons, oatmeal should be a regular part of a healthy diet.

For a dieter, oatmeal can also help you lose weight. The soluble fiber in oatmeal absorbs a large amount of water which slows down the digestive process, making you feel full longer.

TOP SIRTFOODS: 20 FOODS THAT ACTIVATE WEIGHT LOSS.

Sirt foods help signal the body that it should rev up your metabolism and increase muscle mass while you burn fat. Also known as superfoods, the top 20 sirtfoods include the list below. Note that everyone gets excited about the wine and chocolate but your body is actually consistently eating more fiber, more antioxidants, and nutrient-dense foods.

- Kale
- Red wine
- Strawberries
- Onions
- Garlic
- Soy
- Parsley
- Extra virgin olive oil
- Dark chocolate (85% cocoa)
- Matcha green tea
- Buckwheat
- Turmeric
- Walnuts
- Arugula (rocket)
- Bird's eye chili (peppers)
- Lovage (herb)

- Medjool dates
- Red chicory
- Blueberries
- Capers
- Coffee

How to Start:

Week 1 - On the Sirtfood diet means you limit your calorie intake to 1,000 calories a day and drink three Sirtfood green juices throughout the day. The ingredients of a Sirtfood green juice are: Kale, arugula, parsley, celery, including the leaves, half a green apple, the juice of half of a lemon, and matcha green tea (we like. You can have it over ice or add water but don't add plant-based milk or other ingredients not on the list above.

Week 2 - You should increase calories to 1,500 a day and only drink two of the Sirtfood Juices a day, plus have two sirtfood meals each day. Continue on this pattern until you have lost the healthy amount of weight that your body needs to feel your best.

The healthy slow and steady weight loss will add up. If you lose 2 to 3 pounds a week that means you'll have lost 15 pounds in five weeks. Keep in mind that losing weight isn't a fast process and it wouldn't happen overnight, so if you have more than a small amount to lose, just tell yourself that consistency is the key, in order to sustain it over time.

Are Sirtfoods the New Superfoods?

There's no denying that sirtfoods are good for you. They are often high in nutrients and full of healthy plant compounds.

Moreover, studies have associated many of the foods recommended on the Sirtfood Diet with health benefits. For example, eating moderate amounts of dark chocolate with a high cocoa content may lower the risk of heart disease and help fight inflammation. Drinking green tea may reduce the risk of stroke and diabetes and help lower blood pressure.

And turmeric has anti-inflammatory properties that have beneficial effects on the body in general and may even protect against chronic, inflammation-related diseases. In fact, the majority of sirtfoods have demonstrated health benefits in humans. However, evidence on the health benefits of increasing sirtuin protein levels is preliminary. Yet, research in animals and cell lines have shown exciting results.

For example, researchers have found that increased levels of certain sirtuin proteins lead to longer lifespan in yeast, worms and mice. And during fasting or calorie restriction, sirtuin proteins tell the body to burn more fat for energy and improve insulin sensitivity. One study in mice found that increased sirtuin levels led to fat loss. Some evidence suggests that sirtuins may also play a role in reducing inflammation, inhibiting the development of tumors and slowing the development of heart disease and Alzheimer's.

While studies in mice and human cell lines have shown positive results, there have been no human studies examining the effects of increasing sirtuin levels. Therefore, whether increasing sirtuin protein levels in the body will lead to longer lifespan or a lower risk of cancer in humans is unknown. Research is currently underway to develop compounds effective at increasing sirtuin levels in the body. This way, human studies can begin to examine the effects of sirtuins on human health.

Until then, it's not possible to determine the effects of increased sirtuin levels.

Is It Healthy and Sustainable?

Sirtfoods are almost all healthy choices and may even result in some health benefits due to their antioxidant or anti-inflammatory properties. Yet eating just a handful of particularly healthy foods cannot meet all of your body's nutritional needs. The Sirtfood Diet is unnecessarily restrictive and offers no clear, unique health benefits over any other type of diet.

Furthermore, eating only 1,000 calories is typically not recommended without the supervision of a physician. Even eating 1,500 calories per day is excessively restrictive for many people. The diet also requires drinking up to three green juices per day. Although juices can be a good source of vitamins and minerals, they are also a source of sugar and contain almost none of the healthy fiber that whole fruits and vegetables do. What's more, sipping on juice throughout the whole day is a bad idea for both your blood sugar and your teeth.

Not to mention, because the diet is so limited in calories and food choice, it is more than likely deficient in protein, vitamins and minerals, especially during the first phase. Due to the low calorie levels and restrictive food choices, this diet may be difficult to stick to for the entire three weeks. Add that to the high initial costs of having to purchase a juicer, the book and certain rare and expensive ingredients, as well as the time costs of preparing specific meals and juices, and this diet becomes unfeasible and unsustainable for many people.

Safety and Side Effects

Although the first phase of the Sirtfood Diet is very low in calories and nutritionally incomplete, there are no real safety concerns for the average, healthy adult considering the diet's short duration.

Yet for someone with diabetes, calorie restriction and drinking mostly juice for the first few days of the diet may cause dangerous changes in blood sugar levels.

Nevertheless, even a healthy person may experience some side effects, mainly hunger. Eating only 1,000–1,500 calories per day will leave just about anyone feeling hungry, especially if much of what you're consuming is juice, which is low in fiber, a nutrient that helps keep you feeling full. During phase one, you might experience other side effects such as fatigue, lightheadedness and irritability due to the calorie restriction. For the otherwise healthy adult, serious health consequences are unlikely if the diet is followed for only three week

HOW NOT TO LOSE MUSCLE WHILE BURNING FAT?

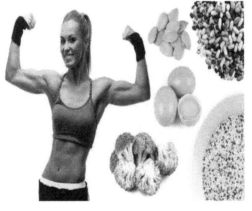 Most people want to know how to build bigger muscles, while burning a large amount of fat at the same time. In fact, some say you can definitely do both at the same time where others deny otherwise.

This has been debated for quite some time now. Well, the answer to this question is yes and no and depends.

You see, you can build bigger muscles and burn fat at the same time. However, if you are using a fat loss exercise workout routine and also at the same time going through a fat loss diet, you will not be able to build a lot of muscles.

You will also burn more fats during your routines if your body possesses more muscles. Well, it is a common impression that more muscles will cause a person to look big and bulky, but this is not always the case.

Bodybuilders are known to have a small amount of body fat while having a huge amount of muscles.

The reason why body builders are able to burn fat and muscles because they do it in phases. It is called periodization in the muscle building world. When body builders build muscles, their diet differs drastically from their exercise routines compared to when they are in the phase of losing fats. These body builders will build mass muscles for several months by segmenting different body part workout routines, as well as lifting heavy weight with low repetitions. It is only that they will change their diet completely from one of building muscle to one which is trying to lose fat. If you have the time, energy and dedication, you may work towards that time of routine, hence, eventually becoming a body builder yourself. But if you just a novice exerciser who just wishes to burn fat and build muscles which are just nice, you can choose a routine and diet which you can burn fat and at the same time, burn a small amount of muscle.

A great way you can approach this to undergo cardio training combined with total body strength training. You see when you perform total body strength training, this will help you to increase your metabolism rate to help you to burn the unwanted fats. When combined with the right type of cardio training, you are on the pathway to successfully burn fats and building bigger muscles at the same time.

Not to forget, your diet will affect your capability to burn fat and muscle too. Consuming quality protein, healthy fats, and complex carbohydrate in a small meal scale 4 - 6 times a day will help you burn more fats because your blood sugar is more constant to help in controlling your appetite.

Tips to build muscle and burn fat

The goal of many body builders is to gain muscles while burning fats. In order to gain muscles, the body needs food and reduction of extraneous activities. While burning fats the body needs much few calories and lots of more tedious cardiovascular exercises. If one wants to embark on a mutual compromise between bulking and cutting typically would result to a compromise outcome. Possibly burning fats without muscle gain or vice versa.

With the advancement of knowledge and understanding the various system of human body and its function, one can apply correct exercise and nutritional intake to better enable one to achieve the goal of increasing muscle mass and losing fat simultaneously.

Here are tips on how to build muscle and burn fats:

1. Engage in cardiovascular exercise

Cardiovascular exercises should be done 3-6 days alternated between longer, slow duration cardio and fast cardio exercise. Walking on a slightly inclined treadmill for 45 minutes is an ideal form of the longer duration cardiovascular exercise, which should be performed on weight training days up to 3x a week. Sprinting outdoors, on a treadmill and/or cycling is an ideal form of fast cardiovascular exercise, which should be done on weight training off days 2-3 times per week.

2. Do weight training

The actual weight training exercises is as important as the timing. It is important to do this exercise in the late afternoon and early evening to allow one to burn fat throughout the day. It is at this time when one will be eating a lower calorie and low carbohydrates diet. Doing exercise too early in the day would halt fat burning for the rest of the day. It should be early in the evening to allow 6 hours interval between weight training session and bedtime. During sleep is the time to drive protein synthesis and replenish glycogen stores. The weight training should be done 3 times a week on alternate days. Each session should consist of heavy basic compound movements with some overlap. Example to it would be chest and back focus on Monday, leg focus on Wednesday, shoulders and arms focus on Friday. All the exercises should be hard, heavy, intense, and cover the entire body.

3. Do a two separate phase of diet.

The diet should be done in two separate phases, the low calorie low carbohydrate portion and the high calorie and high carbohydrate portion. The guidelines would be, all days on weight training off days and half day on weight training days, one should have low calorie diet. Calorie intake of 10-12 times the body weight, consisting of 50% protein, 30 % fat and 20% carbohydrates.

During weight training days, one should have high calorie, high carbohydrate diet. Calorie intake should be 10-12 times the body weight, consisting of 20% protein, 5% fats and 75% carbohydrates. The meal should be consumed in a span of 6-8 hours.

On maintenance phase, calorie intake should be 15 times the body weight, consisting of 50% protein, 30% fat and 20 % carbohydrates.

The weight training and dieting phase do not only burn fats but also put the body to a glycogen-depleted state that heightens insulin sensitivity. By doing so, the body is ready to suck up on all the nutrients delivered during the short-term carbohydrate overfeed. There will be an increase in levels of insulin as the body responds to this overfeeding. Studies have shown that there will be a very small effect on conversion of carbohydrate to fats during massive short-term carbohydrate overfeeding.

4. Take supplements

Taking supplements can help in achieving the required nutritional value to build muscles and reduce fats.

There are several ways to achieve muscle bulk at the same time losing weight. The right combination and timing of diet and exercise is the key. So if one is dreaming to gain muscle and shed off those fats, follow the four tips mentioned above.

It is simply amazing how fast the body will revert to the way it was designed to look when we enact proper nutrition and strength building exercise upon it. In order for a diet to work fast, people must take both halves of the program seriously. In fact, there are countless cases where a 'morbidly obese' person completely changes their diet and starts to do exercises designed to increase muscle mass, resulting in amazing success.

These people, almost without fail, lose the greatest percentage of fat in the first month of the program. Anyone who watches the program, the Biggest Loser, has seen the huge results that the committed contestants achieve in the first three or four weeks of the show.

The body WANTS to be perfect. It is designed to be a lean, tough, survival-driven machine and not a sedentary, fat-storing body.

The body WILL store fat because, according to theorists, human ancestors had to go long periods of time without meat or bountiful food supplies. So, the body learned to store a little for those long migrations and periods of time.

The unfortunate side effect of that human genetic disposition is that now people can choose to eat constantly or get into a rut of snacking constantly. The kinds of diets that work the fastest or those that are primarily built on high-quality, lean protein, good carbohydrates, and healthy fats and oils. Of course, with any recommended diet, drinking more water will do wonders to boost the metabolism and speed up the journey to the desired results.

Eating 5 or 6 smaller meals a day and hitting a specific calorie count per day, while adding strength and muscle building exercise will show the results of our labor within weeks. Normally, a person's face will look noticeably thinner within 5 to 7 days. The double chin seems to be where the body likes to take its stored energy first, visibly speaking.

People looking for diets that work fast and who have a realistic sense of how much work they need to get to their ideal weight are usually people looking to just drop a few extra pounds so they can fit into a dress or swimsuit by the next week or two. For people who need to lose 30 lbs. or more, fast does not mean one or two weeks. Considering that the body of work that must be completed is greater for someone who has not taken in the right foods or has not stuck to an exercise program in years than for someone who has just slacked off for the past couple of weeks.

So, in the case of needing to burn more fat, fast certainly will not equal easy. In order to show real gains within two or three weeks, eating must be taken to a level of perfection and exercise must be done six times per week.

This is not news to anyone, but before putting new kinds of stress on your body, talk to a doctor and get the okay to do so. Taking on a workout program like Shaun T's Insanity or P90X after 10 years of bodily abuse by diet, smoking, and laziness could do damage in the short-term. Some people will need to warm up with lighter workouts, but the diet still must be absolutely perfect if the gains they are looking for are to be accomplished in a relatively short period of time. In the end, the diets that work the fastest are the ones that only allow the three healthy food pillars mentioned above, involve muscle-building exercise, and increase the amount of water the person drinks.

You have been bombarded lately by so many ads online or in TV trying to suggest the only diets that work for you. Yet, none of these guaranteed weight loss plans did not produce any result or you have lost couple pounds, but not for long.

Now you sitting back behind your computer trying to look for another fad diets that will give you the answer you've been searching for: What are the diets that work?

To be very honest with you is that the diets that are promoted are all garbage. Yes. Garbage. None of those fad diet do not work. It might start making sense to you why you could not lose weight. Also you should know that all those diets are the cause of you Yo-Yo Dieting, losing fat and gaining more in couple of weeks, being cranky and stressful etc.

As hard as it is to believe diets are nothing else that the way you eat! So if you are going to McDonnald every day, you are probably on McBurger diet. If you go to your nearest Pizza shop, you are on a pizza diet. Those are not diets that will help you to lose fat and reveal your six-pack.

Then you have diets that have all components and food groups like chicken, beans and rice. Or sweet potato with broccoli and char-coal grilled chicken breast.

What these diets contain is protein (needed to build muscles), carbohydrates (needed to feed your brain and give you source of energy) and vegetables (filled with nutrients, minerals and fiber to feed every cell of your body and help you digest better).

And at last you have the above mentioned diets that scream at you when watching TV, listening the radio or browsing online search engines. Most of them will make you lose weight, but it won't be fat loss but major muscle loss. You really can't afford to lose muscles. Because what you will gain back will be more fat. You will completely change your body composition and that is what will make it much harder to lose fat in the future.

So stop chasing those diets that will remove either proteins, carbs or fibers out of your diet. Your perfect diets that work for you should have all food groups and therefore basic building blocks for body. Nothing more, nothing less.

Many people don't get a clear idea of how to choose the diet that works for them. This is usually because they feel misled or do not clearly understand the complicated language used in diet books. To make things simpler, let's set categories of lifestyles where you could recognize your way of living so that you start losing pounds now.

Are you someone who performs strenuous jobs daily and stay in the sun? If yes, it is important to know that a healthy diet is different for you too. People who make a lot of effort spend calories while at work. A diet with a higher rate of energy in the form of fats, protein and carbohydrates is acceptable in this case, however, it is also very important to consume water plentifully. Fruits and vegetables are also important.

Are you the type of person who does his/her work sitting? The form of energy you will be using in that case will surely also make you feel as tired too. This is because you need some fresh air. It is very important to take plenty of fruits and vegetables in this case as they are essential to remedy your tired nerves. Fats should really be avoided and protein foods should be taken in small quantities only.

Are you recovering from a long sickness or did you have an accident and got your bones broken? When something is wrong in your body, your body cells and tissues usually get affected and make you feel ill. You get feverish or rashes because your body had been undergoing a war with germs. This may require you to do a lot of cleaning up and replacing the dead cells. For this, food rich in protein and vitamins and minerals are very important. If you have fractures, it does not really mean you're sick. But food rich in calcium is important to build your bones anew!

So how do you find diets that work?

Simply these diets should not tell you to eat less and starve yourselves. They should not tell you to eat less carbs, no protein, no vegetables. They can't drastically lower your daily calorie intake and they should not sell you on some miracle pills and do nothing.

Only you can choose what diet is best for you. You just need to get more educated about foods, exercise and stress reduction. Remember, your diet is the one you feel fantastic about. No chores or drudgery there. Then you know that you have found diets that work for you.

There are people in the world today who want to have an attractive look as well as nice figure. These people spend a fortune on diets that can help them lose weight. There are a lot of sites that can suggest meals or diets that "work" when one wants to lose weight. But many of these sites are best left avoided since the diet programs they suggest are rather ambiguous and could even jeopardize your plans to shed that excess weight you have. A recent study has shown that Americans are spending more or less $70 billion dollars a year when it comes to dieting and losing weight and the figure goes up annually.

Real diets that work when it comes to losing weight and having an attractive figure include those espoused by professionals such as dietitians, doctors and nutritionists among others. In making preparations for charting a diet, elements like age, preference in food, gender, work and so forth are to be considered. The diets being planned for the chart can be varied for every meal. For example, you can have some fruit as a snack while you can have some vegetables along with pasta for lunch, as these have low levels of fat. The same can be said for your breakfast as well as the dinner you'll be having. Foods such as fruits and vegetables are a very sustainable source of energy. In time, you can develop a reduced liking to something like fast food.

In case you want to build up your muscle mass, there are also diets that work on that. What you need to do so is to have high protein meals. These include meat such as chicken, beef and turkey, fish as well as free-range eggs. Foods having high protein content increase the feeling of being "full" and, in time also lower your craving to overeat.

In addition to the ones mentioned, you should also seek professional advice since this can help you plan balanced diets in more detail in addition to helping you get motivated. These professionals know how to prepare diets that work depending on what sort of activities you do and what sort of food you like.

Diets that work are prepared with losing weight as well as maintaining a body that's fit as well as healthy. What's vital to a diet that succeeds is in having an air of positivity when it comes to living life as well as the conviction to change the way you eat.

An easy diet plan

Are you tired and want to lose those unwanted inches and pounds that you have gained over the last couple of years. All because you were feeling old, unattractive and not that interested in anything at all. Well let me put your mind to rest, because you are not alone. There are hundreds of people online right now that feel like you do, and doing the same thing you are. Their looking to find a diet that will work and provide all the information they need to make an informative decision.

There are a number of diets that work well, very well. You might have seen the show, "The Biggest Loser" on TV. That Diet or Weight Loss Plan works very, very well. People lose and incredible amount of weight each week. Double digit weight losses are very common for most of the contestants. That would be unhealthy for most but those contestants are closely monitored and fed special diets. Most important is they have so much excess water and fat build up that it is healthier for them to get rid of it at that rate. They are put on a exercise program that pushes them to vomit and tears.

Most of us can't afford or don't have the luxury of having that much time to go to a health resort for that kind of weight loss program. That's too bad because most of us need to be educated on the importance of proper nutrition and good fitness.

The contestants on the biggest loser have that advantage. They are fully examined and are sat down at told there realistic age of their body. They are shown what their organs look like compared to a normal organ. They are shown why they are going to die at a much earlier age than a normal life span. That gives them a good start on the mindset needed to go through a serious weight loss plan and then to continue to diet. The other half of the mindset is they are asked to write down all the reasons they want to get healthy and live a long life. Once a person has good reasons to live longer and is shown the reasons why that won't happen the mindset is in place. That is an important part to a long lasting lifestyle change. Not every diet works for everybody. In fact, it is not always the diet that does not work. Certain diets work differently for different people. Diets that work for one may not work for another. Everyone is different, and all the pills, powders, liquids and systems, programs and plans all work differently, too. Some pills will make you very shaky. This is due to the caffeine in them. The weight only comes off when you are putting in the effort. If you are not trying or you are just taking the pills and hoping for the best. No, of course it is not going to work, you cannot lose five pounds in five days without trying. There is a lot of work that has to take place in order to lose weight.

Eating healthy food and excise is a much better way to lose weight, this is how the revolutionary diet plan, Strip That Fat fits into your life. I consider this a true diet plan, you eat real food 4 - 5 times a day, so you are not starving yourself. And with this diet plan you get what is called the Strip That Fat Diet Generator software which you enter into the generator, the foods you like to eat, then it sets up a diet plan that you follow. When you what to make changes within your diet plan just enter into the diet generator what you want and again it will create another plan for you. It also prints a shopping list to help make it easier to get what you need, in order to follow your diet plan.

It also comes with a guide that explains everything you need to know about dieting, like what works and why, what does not work and the reasons why they don't. The complete Strip That Fat Diet Plan and Generator and all the information you could possible want to assist you along the way to your weight loss goal. There must be some form of exercise in order to lose that unwanted fat. A brisk walk every day is a great way to start, increasing your heart rate to the fat burning zone for at least 15 minutes to start. Then as you get comfortable with that you can start to build 20, 30 minutes, increasing slowly. You can strip those unwanted ponds and inches right off in no time at all. There are very few diets or weight loss plans that make it simple by teaching proper nutrition without making drastic lifestyle changes. Also teach simple exercises that slowly tone your body instead of drastic lifestyle changes of daily vigorous workouts. If you try to change your lifestyle too quickly in too many different ways it usually will fail. That is what studies show. A plan that "Works" is one that you can live with for life. That is a good healthy weight loss plan or diet that works.

So if you're looking for one that works, do some research and read what the plans intentions are. See if it teaches you all about nutrition and lets you eat the foods you like to eat. See if it is something you can live with for long term, not just short term. Why pay a lot of money for something that is not going to last long? Why suffer for a short term loss of weight? If you learn how to lose weight properly it isn't real difficult. Weight goes on one pound at a time over a long period of time and that is how it should come off.

If your definition of "works" is just lose a few pounds then quit and gain it back then start all over again, take your pick of plans, they all "Work".

HOW TO IMPROVE YOUR ENERGY-BOOSTING EFFECT (EBE)

We all lead such hectic lives that being constantly tired or lacking energy can seem almost normal for many people. Just getting by can take up most of our energy, leaving little left to use to work towards our goals or building our ideal life.

It seems that most successful people have high energy levels. There may be exceptions, but I think it's fair to say that there's probably not that many examples of people who are constantly tired or exhausted, or burned out, achieving and sustaining high levels of success.

So what can we do to increase our energy levels?
Getting enough sleep, relaxing and taking time off when you don't work at all, are the most obvious essentials to maintaining energy levels.

It will also help if we understand the different types of energy we use in our lives. There is more than one type of energy. The main types of energy are physical, emotional and mental. Although these are distinctly different, they are closely related and interdependent.

Physical Energy

Physical energy is the most basic type of energy. This is the energy that's used in manual labour. People who are involved in this kind of work usually need to eat substantial quantities of food just to sustain themselves. In many cases, at the end of each day they will have little energy left over for anything more than relaxing and sleeping so they can rebuild their strength in preparation for the next day. This is the situation for much of the world's population, particularly in developing countries.

Fortunately, due to automation, labour saving inventions, computers etc many of us no longer have to work as hard physically as previous generations did. More people than ever are employed in knowledge based roles requiring little or no physical effort.

Emotional Energy

Emotional energy is the energy that allows us to experience happiness, joy, love, excitement and many other emotions, both good and bad. This is the energy that gives us our enthusiasm and our love of life, and allows us to have fun. Many of our actions are driven, in varying degrees, by our emotional energy. Our emotions can have a great impact on our overall energy levels.

When you are with friends and loved ones and are happy, excited or having fun, you will usually find that you have plenty you energy and feel great. This type of interaction with others not only boosts energy levels, but is good for overall health and resistance to illness.

Unsurprisingly, negative emotions have the opposite effect. If you are feeling angry, upset, depressed, frustrated or stressed, for example, you'll find your energy levels depleted and your resistance weak. If you keep feeling this way for extended periods, you'll eventually burn out altogether. If you can maximise positive emotions and maintain an overall optimistic outlook you'll find that you have more energy that you can put to good use in other areas of your life.

Mental Energy

The other type of energy is mental energy. As many of us now work in knowledge based roles, we use a lot of this type of energy on a daily basis. This is the energy of creativity, decision making, writing, reading, learning new information and much more. Most of us now rely on our mental energy to survive.

How effectively we use our mental energy will ultimately decide how successful we are in our lives. It is our mental energy, through our thought processes, that determines our values and goals and the actions we take, which ultimately determine what we make of our lives.

How well we maximise the use of our mental energy and powers will be a major factor determining how successful and happy our lives turn out.

Negative Energy

One common setback to success is burning up energy in destructive ways. Although most of us don't now engage in much hard physical work, many of us waste huge amounts of emotional energy. This can take many forms. It could be something a common as having a generally negative outlook on life. There are many other examples, such as being over sensitive or easily upset, or being prone to emotional outbursts of anger or even violence.

Negative emotions can massively drain energy levels, in fact a five minute outburst of anger uses about as much energy as eight hours of mental work.

Being at your best mentally depends on being at your best emotionally. Keeping calm, not letting things bother you, and maintaining a positive mental outlook can make a huge difference to your emotional state, which will boost your mental and physical energy. So will ensuring you get enough sleep, taking time to relax and taking regular breaks where you forget your work altogether. These can be the critical difference between being always tired, highly stressed or constantly on edge, and enjoying a successful, rewarding and happy life.

How to increase your energy levels

Do you feel you are performing at your best? Do you spring out of bed in the morning, excited and ready for the opportunities your day presents? Imagine for a moment you are the proud owner of a champion, thorough bred horse worth in excess of one million dollars.

As the owner of this prized purebred, would you let him stay up half the night, drink coffee and booze, smoke cigarettes and eat junk food? What about your $10 dog? Your $5 cat?

You see, most people treat their own bodies with less care than they would treat a $5 cat. If you did own a horse worth one million dollars, you would hire a nutritionist to make sure his diet was exactly right, you would also ensure he was getting his regular massages and spine alignment treatments; the best supplementation; you would have the best trainer in the country; an air-conditioned barn in the summer time, a steam-heated one in the winter time a million dollar investment. And here you have this BILLION dollar body.

When Was Your Last 100,000km Service?

The problem is that we expect our body will just do what it is supposed to do no matter what kind of treatment it receives. We often take better care of our car ensuring it gets regular service, appropriate maintenance and oil changes in the necessary intervals, but when it comes to our own bodies, the service is usually below par.

Our bodies have amazing coping, self-correcting mechanisms. It is able to handle, quite literally, long-term abuse, without much complaint for long periods. It waits patiently to be treated well with only slow and gradual decline in health and vitality, until the day it decides: That's it, I've had enough!--only then we start paying attention.

The First Sign, Help Is Needed!

The first aspect of our health that starts to signal a need for 'help' relates to our general wellbeing and vitality: Our energy levels. We often misinterpret the body's needs or simply ignore them--what the body really is asking for when it lacks energy is for us to take care: sleep more, eat well, exercise, re-hydrate. But instead of that we end up giving it lots of coffee, energy drinks, sugar and telling ourselves to 'snap out of it' as we go on abusing it. That is not a smart long-term strategy. In fact, it only leads to one thing: Disease.

How Do I Make It All Better?

The solution is to STOP and go back to basics. However, before you change anything it is vital to assess where you are at and where you would like to be. In my practice we have some fancy machines to do that, we also take our patients through very comprehensive and detailed assessments to ensure we are both clear about the starting point (a baseline is paramount), however one of the tools we use which is available to you right now is a simple question:--What are you energy levels on a scale of 0-10 10=excellent)? Once you have the answer to this question you can start implementing the following suggestions to substantially increase your energy levels. In fact, a 300% energy increase is very realistic. When a person is operating at 2/10 and for the time, that is their 100%, it doesn't take long, when applying the tips below to increase levels to a generous and vibrant 8/10. Keep going and you will ACE it!

Practical Steps For Energy Maximization

Once you know where you are at, you can measure your progress as you go along. Here are 7 tips that will transform your energy levels and vitality within one week of diligent application. The catch is that you need to keep your practice up for at least 28 days to see the full benefit of your new investment in yourself.

1. Clean Up Your Diet

Let go of all junk. Base your meals on fresh, organic, seasonal produce (fruits and vegetables) and good quality protein (e.g. eggs, quark, chicken, beef, lamb, kangaroo, venison etc). The less unprocessed your foods the better. Avoid canned and pre-prepared meals.

2. Have Protein For Breakfast

If you could only do ONE thing on this list--this would have to be it. Eating good quality protein for breakfast is one of the only things that will ensure you do not get any energy slumps in the afternoon. So try poached or boiled eggs; fruit smoothie with quark; fruit with cottage cheese or quark; toast with sardines or (flaked) grilled salmon.

3. Eat Every 3 Hours

This will ensure your energy is leveled during the day. Ensuring your moods, focus, concentration are all optimum. This is easier than you think. Just divide up what you would normally eat in one sitting for a meal into two. Your digestive system will have an easier job and your energy levels will skyrocket.

4. What To Drink And What Not To Drink?

When cells become dehydrated, they don't perform the metabolic processed necessary to ensure proper detoxification and optimum energy. So ensuring you have a large 2L bottle with you or a jug on your desk--knowing that by the end of the day the whole thing needs to be finished will be your best way forward. Also ensure your have a good quality water filter for this purpose; toxins found in unfiltered or poorly filtered water will damage your health. You want to make sure your filter is as fine as 1 micron or more.

In addition, be sure to avoid (or at least drastically cut down on the consumption of) coffee and alcohol, as well as sugary and energy drinks including undiluted fruit juices. These substances dramatically disturb your blood sugar levels and energy balance. Coffee and alcohol are also very dehydrating, also depleting the body of essential nutrients necessary to ensure optimum energy.

5. Get Enough And Quality Sleep

If your body is not resting sufficiently at night--no matter what you do during the day, your energy levels will not improve. Start by planning your life around getting enough sleep, not the other way around. Budget for 7-9 hours of sleep time each night. If you are having problems, sleeping you will see that by implementing all the previous suggestions this should improve. Alternatively, seek help; there are many effective natural tools you can implement for a better night's sleep.

6. Exercise & Nutritional support

Being active is the best way to balance your blood sugar levels. Also when you exercise your body releases endorphins which are feel good chemicals that also boost your energy levels. There are so many benefits to exercise, if you are not doing it,you are missing out! Aim to do something for at least 40 minutes, no less 4 days per week. Build up to this slowly if necessary--but just get out there!

7. Spinal Alignment & Nutritional Support

It is all very well to want to build a house, but if you are missing key building materials, it is not going to happen--no matter how much you want it. This is the role of nutrients in the body. Unfortunately when the body becomes depleted, diet alone is not sufficient to correct the problem. Each individual has different requirement and an assessment of your needs, as well as what other supplements or medicines you are currently taking is really important before embarking on any new supplementation. Resolving depleted or deficient states in your body can make a world of difference to your energy levels!

Another key aspect of energy is spinal your spine health and alignment--this also hinges on appropriate nutritional markers, however ensuring proper blood flow to tissues, and key body parts such as the brain is essential for energy and for this you just cannot go passed a good chiropractor or osteopath.

Keep these up and your billion dollar asset will reward you with bountiful energy, remarkable vitality and robust wellbeing. What more could you want?

The Sirtfood Juice

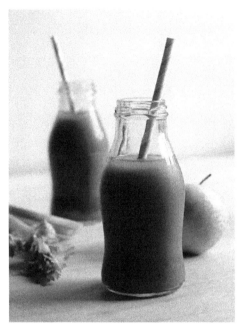

A good way to start is with The Sirtfood Juice – so we've thrown in the recipe for this to start you off as a bonus extra. The book advises drinking 3 juices and adding 1 meal for the first 3 days, then 2 juices, 2 meals for the next 4.Sirtfood Green Juice (serves 1)

Ingredients:

- 2 large handfuls (75g) kale
- a large handful (30g) rocket
- a very small handful (5g) flat-leaf parsley
- a very small handful (5g) lovage leaves (optional)
- 2–3 large stalks (150g) green celery, including its leaves
- ½ medium green apple
- juice of ½ lemon
- ½ level tsp matcha green tea

Instructions:

Mix the greens (kale, rocket, parsley and lovage, if using) together, then juice them. We find juicers can really differ in their efficiency at juicing leafy vegetables and you may need to re-juice the remnants before moving on to the other ingredients. The goal is to end up with about 50ml of juice from the greens.

Now juice the celery and apple.You can peel the lemon and put it through the juicer as well, but we find it much easier to simply squeeze the lemon by hand into the juice. By this stage, you should have around 250ml of juice in total, perhaps slightly more.It is only when the juice is made and ready to serve that you add the matcha green tea.

Pour a small amount of the juice into a glass, then add the matcha and stir vigorously with a fork or teaspoon. We only use matcha in the first two drinks of the day as it contains moderate amounts of caffeine (the same content as a normal cup of tea). For people not used to it, it may keep them awake if drunk late.Once the matcha is dissolved add the remainder of the juice.

Give it a final stir, then your juice is ready to drink. Feel free to top up with plain water, according to taste.

Aromatic chicken breast with kale and red onions and a tomato and chilli salsa (serves 1)

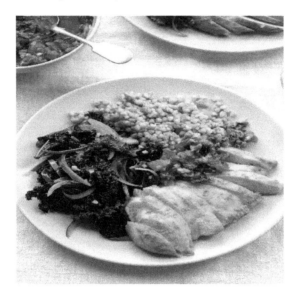

Ingredients:

- 120g skinless, boneless chicken breast
- 2 tsp ground turmeric
- juice of ¼ lemon
- 1 tbsp extra virgin olive oil
- 50g kale, chopped
- 20g red onion, sliced
- 1 tsp chopped fresh ginger
- 50g buckwheat
- For the salsa
- 130g tomato (about 1)
- 1 bird's eye chilli, finely chopped

- 1 tbsp capers, finely chopped
- 5g parsley, finely chopped
- Juice of ¼ lemon

Instructions:

To make the salsa, remove the eye from the tomato and chop it very finely, taking care to keep as much of the liquid as possible. Mix with the chilli, capers, parsley and lemon juice. You could put everything in a blender but the end result is a little different.

Heat the oven to 220°C/gas 7. Marinate the chicken breast in 1 teaspoon of the turmeric, the lemon juice and a little oil. Leave for 5–10 minutes.Heat an ovenproof frying pan until hot, then add the marinated chicken and cook for a minute or so on each side, until pale golden, then transfer to the oven (place on a baking tray if your pan isn't ovenproof) for 8–10 minutes or until cooked through. Remove from the oven, cover with foil and leave to rest for 5 minutes before serving.

Meanwhile, cook the kale in a steamer for 5 minutes. Fry the red onions and the ginger in a little oil, until soft but not coloured, then add the cooked kale and fry for another minute.Cook the buckwheat according to the packet instructions with the remaining teaspoon of turmeric. Serve alongside the chicken, vegetables and salsa.

Sirtfood bites (makes 15-20 bites)

Ingredients:

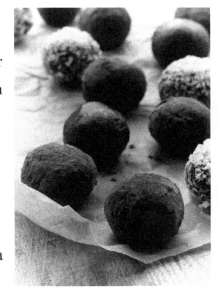

- 120g walnuts
- 30g dark chocolate (85 per cent cocoa solids), broken into pieces; or cocoa nibs
- 250g Medjool dates, pitted
- 1 tbsp cocoa powder
- 1 tbsp ground turmeric
- 1 tbsp extra virgin olive oil
- the scraped seeds of 1 vanilla pod or 1 tsp vanilla extract
- 1–2 tbsp water

Instructions:

Place the walnuts and chocolate in a food processor and process until you have a fine powder.

Add all the other ingredients except the water and blend until the mixture forms a ball. You may or may not have to add the water depending on the consistency of the mixture – you don't want it to be too sticky.

Using your hands, form the mixture into bite-sized balls and refrigerate in an airtight container for at least 1 hour before eating them. You could roll some of the balls in some more cocoa or desiccated coconut to achieve a different finish if you like. They will keep for up to 1 week in your fridge.

Asian king prawn stir-fry with buckwheat noodles (serves 1)

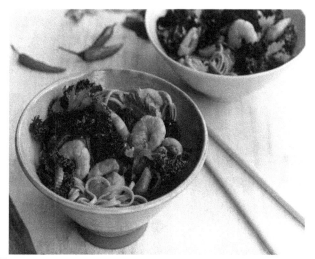

Ingredients:

- 150g shelled raw king prawns, deveined
- 2 tsp tamari (you can use soy sauce if you are not avoiding gluten)
- 2 tsp extra virgin olive oil
- 75g soba (buckwheat noodles)
- 1 garlic clove, finely chopped
- 1 bird's eye chilli, finely chopped
- 1 tsp finely chopped fresh ginger

- 20g red onions, sliced
- 40g celery, trimmed and sliced
- 75g green beans, chopped
- 50g kale, roughly chopped
- 100ml chicken stock
- 5g lovage or celery leaves

Instructions:

Heat a frying pan over a high heat, then cook the prawns in 1 teaspoon of the tamari and 1 teaspoon of the oil for 2–3 minutes. Transfer the prawns to a plate. Wipe the pan out with kitchen paper, as you're going to use it again.

Cook the noodles in boiling water for 5–8 minutes or as directed on the packet. Drain and set aside.

Meanwhile, fry the garlic, chilli and ginger, red onion, celery, beans and kale in the remaining oil over a medium–high heat for 2–3 minutes. Add the stock and bring to the boil, then simmer for a minute or two, until the vegetables are cooked but still crunchy.

Add the prawns, noodles and lovage/celery leaves to the pan, bring back to the boil then remove from the heat and serve.

Strawberry buckwheat tabouleh

Ingredients:

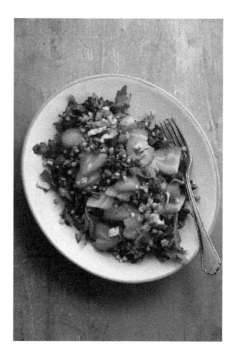

- 50g buckwheat
- 1 tbsp ground turmeric
- 80g avocado
- 65g tomato
- 20g red onion
- 25g Medjool dates, pitted
- 1 tbsp capers
- 30g parsley
- 100g strawberries, hulled
- 1 tbsp extra virgin olive oil
- juce of ½ lemon
- 30g rocket

Instructions:

Cook the buckwheat with the turmeric according to the packet instructions. Drain and keep to one side to cool.

Finely chop the avocado, tomato, red onion, dates, capers and parsley and mix with the cool buckwheat. Slice the strawberries and gently mix into the salad with the oil and lemon juice. Serve on a bed of rocket.

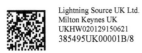

Lightning Source UK Ltd.
Milton Keynes UK
UKHW020129150621
385495UK00001B/8

9 781802 782233